All About Arthritis

Find Updated Causes, Symptoms, Diagnostic Tests, New Alternative Treatments, Cures and Breakthroughs

Michael P. Angelillo M.D.

iUniverse, Inc.
New York Bloomington

iUniverse books may be ordered through booksellers or by contacting:

iUniverse
1663 Liberty Drive
Bloomington, IN 47403
www.iuniverse.com
1-800-Authors (1-800-288-4677)

Because of the dynamic nature of the Internet, any Web addresses or links contained in this book may have changed since publication and may no longer be valid. The views expressed in this work are solely those of the author and do not necessarily reflect the views of the publisher, and the publisher hereby disclaims any responsibility for them.

ISBN: 978-1-4401-7460-5 (sc)
ISBN: 978-1-4401-7461-2 (ebook)

Printed in the United States of America

iUniverse rev. date: 09/16/09

Dedication

To my three children, Michael, Patrick and Leah...

This book is dedicated to my children who are my greatest accomplishment, pride and joy. They have inspired me in all aspects of my life !

INTRODUCTION

Arthritis is the most common cause of disability in the United States which limits the activities of 46 million adults and 300,000 children. Arthritis may affect many people, but thanks to intensive research over the past several years, we now know more on how to handle arthritis. There are many different forms of arthritis and each has a different cause. Most all types of arthritis feature pain and inflammation. Arthritis can be secondary to other diseases. There are certain diseases that can also mimic arthritis.

As an expert in the field of Rheumatology with over 25 years treating patients in private practice I have written this book which will give you, the reader new and informative information about arthritis, it's causes and symptoms. Diagnostic test will be discussed to reveal various forms of arthritis. Various new treatments to help alleviate the symptoms of arthritis including natural remedies will be fully discussed.

New information regarding foods that can trigger or aggravate arthritic symptoms will be revealed to avoid and things you can do for yourself to stop the progression of arthritis will be explained using my experience and knowledge over a proven 25 year career.

In treating arthritis today there have been many breakthroughs in diagnosis and treatment which patients may not be aware of. This is unfortunate because the delay in treatment or diagnosis could substantially delay the outcome for individual results.

Before reading this book ask yourself, "why shouldn't I know or do everything possible to help myself treat my arthritis so I can help myself feel better!" That is the question that you will have answered after reading this book.

Contents

CHAPTER 1

WHAT IS ARTHRITIS ?

In most cases, arthritis is a natural part of aging, and develops over a lifetime of the use of our joints. The word arthritis, literally means joint inflammation, which is derived from the Greek word "arthros" (joint) and "itis" means (inflammation), and it's major symptom is joint pain. Although the same group of ailments is sometimes called rheumatism, we will call it arthritis in this book. Many people confuse arthritis as a single disease. Arthritis is actually a "catch all term" used to classify a group of more than 100 conditions.

We now know that arthritis can affect any age and comes in various forms. What is common to all types of arthritis is that they can all affect the musculoskeletal system (muscles and bones) and can affect specific joints. There are many related conditions but when talking about arthritis we talk about related joint problems including pain, stiffness, inflammation and the end result in actual damage to the joints and the structures around them.

Arthritis pain varies considerably in severity. It may come and go, which is called episodic pain, or it may be chronic, meaning you will feel it all the time. If this occurs it can lead to joint weakness, instability and deformities. When these joint deformities occur it interferes with the most basic daily tasks such as walking, cutting food, brushing your teeth, using tools, climbing stairs etc.

To classify arthritis you must understand that arthritis can affect the whole entire body. If this occurs these diseases can cause damage to organs including the heart, lungs, kidneys, skin and blood vessels. It is important to understand that when this happens the affected area or organ can present as an initial problem, often confusing your doctor. Commonly most arthritis conditions can affect muscles and joints.

Because of the related conditions which arthritis can be associated with it has caused the United States more than 125 billion per year in medical care and expenses like lost wages and production. An important fact as the population is getting older and people with arthritis and related conditions are expanding. This poses a growing concern for treatment and the urgency to find related cures as soon as possible.

CHAPTER 2

OSTEOARTHRITIS

Today we know there are more than 100 different types of arthritis. Osteoarthritis is by far the most common types of arthritis which affect adults. Another term used for this term is Degenerative Joint Disease. Osteoarthritis is considered a non-inflammatory disorder of movable joints. It strikes more than half of the people over the age of 65 and 80% of those over 75 years old.

Osteoarthritis occurs when your cartilage in your joints wear out over time. The joints affected by this disease is usually your hands, hips, knees and spine. Osteoarthritis can affect one joint at a time or several joints at a time. Over time the joints become worse. There is no cure to date but there are steps you can take to gain control over your pain which I will discuss in this chapter.

The first symptom to develop is pain from the affected joint or joints. You may experience tenderness in the joint affected when you apply light pressure over that joint. Another common symptom of osteoarthritis is joint stiffness either when you have a period of inactivity like in the morning. It may be hard to flex or bend the joint too. Over time you may feel like a griddy sensation in the joint or grinding. Swelling can occur in any joint affected and over time bone spurs appear as hard lumps around the joint.

Osteoarthritis occurs when the cartilage that cushion the ends of bone wear out over time. When the cartilage wears out you may be left with bone rubbing against bone. At this stage of damage your joints will become very painful.

There are many factors that predispose you to develop osteoarthritis. One factor is age. People under the age of 40 rarely develop osteoarthritis. Did you know that women are more likely to develop osteoarthritis? We now know that people who had sport injuries when they were young are more prone to develop osteoarthritis. If you were born with defective cartilage or malformed joints you have an increased risk to develop osteoarthritis. Obese people put excess stress or weight on there joints causing them to be at higher risk.

If you suspect that you are suffering from these symptoms see your doctor and he will confirm this diagnosis with certain tests and X-rays. When the doctor does his X-rays images reveal a narrow space in the joint which means that the cartilage is wearing down. Another finding is that the bone affected has bone spurs around it. Your doctor may want to perform certain other specific blood tests to rule out other forms of arthritis. When fluid is in your joint your doctor may want to take the fluid out for analysis. This procedure which is done in the office is called an arthrocentesis procedure. If a diagnosis is complicated or not clear your doctor may want to insert a camera in your joint. This procedure is called an arthroscopy. By doing this the doctor can actually see the inside of your joint and determine what's causing your pain.

A very real complication of osteoarthritis is disability. Joint pain and stiffness may become severe enough to make getting through the day impossible. When the pain is too severe and you are not able to perform your daily activities it may be time for a joint replacement, either total or partial.

Because my practice in Rheumatology was directly located across the street from a retirement center I was fortunate enough to treat many cases of osteoarthritis in the community. My treatments for osteoarthritis were as follows. If you were experiencing pain in your joint, rest it for approximately 12 hours. Take a break every hour for 10 minutes helped significantly. You should also get regular exercise, walking, swimming with your doctor's approval. Avoid exercising tender, injured or swollen joints. If you develop pain stop. New pain that lasts after exercising means that you've overdone it. Lose weight! Being overweight or obese increases the stress on your joints. The use of heat or cold can relieve pain in your joints. You can soothe your painful joints with heat using a heating pad, hot water bottle or by taking a warm bath. You can use ice packs to relieve muscle spasms and help reduce the pain. Always be careful not to use ice packs if you suffer from poor circulation. To reduce pain and increase the range of motion in your joints you can ask your doctor for a referral to a physical therapist. It is important that the physical therapist that you use create an individualized program which will help you specifically. One of the other modalities that I have prescribed as a rheumatologist is the use of an occupational therapist. An occupational therapist will help you discover ways to do everyday tasks without putting extra stress on your joints. An example is using a special shower seat to relieve the pain on your knees getting in and out of the shower. Creams and gels available at the drug store may provide some relief in your joints. Pain creams usually work better in the smaller joint of the hands because the medicine penetrates through the skin into the joints. When you are in the need to take the pressure off a joint then a brace for support could be prescribed by your doctor. I always suggest to join the Arthritis Foundation for classes on pain management and to get tips on how to manage your arthritis.

Medications may be useful for moderate arthritic pain. By taking Acetaminophen (Tylenol) you can relieve pain but not inflammation. Because Acetaminophen can be bought over the counter patients often neglect to tell their doctor. This medicine can cause liver damage if taken regularly. Nonsteroidal anti-inflammatory drugs called NSAIDs can reduce pain and inflammation. Some are over the counter like Advil or Motrin. Others are by prescription like Celebrex. NSAIDs have a higher risks when used all the time. Side effects include ringing in your ears, gastric ulcers, cardiovascular problems, gastrointestinal bleeding, liver and kidney damage.

When patients suffer from severe osteoarthritis in addition to the above mentioned treatments one can be prescribed stronger pain pills. Codiene has been prescribed as Darvon which may give relief. Be aware of the risk factor for dependence and side effect profile. Side effects of these medications include nausea, constipation, and sleepiness. Cortisone injections may relieve pain in your joints. It is not clear how or why corticosteroids injections work in people with osteoarthritis. It is now known that repeated cortisone injections in a specific joint over a specific time can cause damage to that specific joint. Hyaluronic acid derivatives or what is known as Hyalgan, or Synvisc may offer pain relief by giving the knee a cushioning effect between the cartilage. These medications are similar to what you have in your knee. Because these medications are similar to rooster combs if you are sensitive to birds, feathers or eggs you should not undergo these injections. Notify your doctor! After administration of these particular injections relief may last for months.

When the pain or discomfort is too great and your osteoarthritis is making it too difficult to perform your daily activities of living, knee surgery or joint replacement surgery (arthroplasty) can be performed. This takes place when a surgeon removes your damaged joint surface and replaces it with either plastic or metal device called prostheses. Today the hip and knee joints are most commonly replaced. Other joints can be replaced today and can last up to 20 years. Surgeons now have the ability to realign bones in younger people who cannot have replacement surgery because of their age. This procedure is called osteotomy. Surgeons also have the capability to fuse bones together which is called arthrodesis. This helps to increase stability and reduce pain. In this type of procedure mobility is lost but the pain is relieved.

The key to manage your pain and disability also is your overall attitude. I have seen in my clinical practice over 25 years a better overall outcome with patients with positive attitudes. I have had patients go to hypnosis, guided imagery, deep breathing techniques, and muscle relaxation exercises to help there overall picture. Also know your limitations. Rest when you are tired. There are new treatments for osteoarthritis which I have left in my last chapter of this book. Further discussion about new treatments and breakthroughs are in the last chapter.

CHAPTER 3

RHEUMATOID ARTHRITIS

Rheumatoid Arthritis causes joint pain and damage. This type of arthritis is inflammatory. When the arthritis affects the lining of your joints which is called the synovium it can cause achy type of pain. If this type of inflammation continues it causes deformities of the joints that it affects. Rheumatoid Arthritis can affect children and when it does it is call Juvenile Rheumatoid Arthritis. Rheumatoid Arthritis is three times more common in women than men and can occur between the ages of 40 and 60. Although there is no cure for this type of arthritis with proper treatment you can manage and further protect your joints and live a productive life with this type of arthritis.

There are many symptoms of rheumatoid arthritis.

Most commonly are joint pain and swelling. Joints that are tender to the touch are the joints that are most inflamed. Weight loss, fever, morning stiffness longer than 30 minutes can occur. When you suffer from rheumatoid arthritis you can develop firm bumps on your arms which are called rheumatoid nodules.

Early rheumatoid arthritis usually causes problems in several joints at the same time. The wrists, ankles, hands, and feet are usually affected first. In my office in clinical practice it was common to see flare ups, periods of increased activity with alternating periods of inactivity.

It is now proven in research that the red blood cells in your body play a role in causing the synovium to become inflamed. This inflammation causes release of proteins which over years cause the synovium to thicken. The proteins can also damage the cartilage, bone, tendons and ligaments near your joint. When this occurs the joint can become damaged.

Today we do not know what causes rheumatoid arthritis

but a combination of your gene factors, smoking, and viruses are said to be the main factors. When your doctor suspects you of having rheumatoid arthritis he will do some testing on you. Blood tests are essential like erythrocyte sedimentation rate also called ESR, which indicates inflammation in your body. Testing for rheumatoid factor in your blood will determine if these antibodies are present in your blood. Another blood test used is called anti-cyclic citrullinated peptide also called anti-CCP. If these are found in your blood they have a correlation with an increase in joint damage you may experience. Your doctor may want to take joint fluid out to exam it for rheumatoid arthritis. X-rays may be warranted to evaluate the extent or to monitor the condition. Having rheumatoid arthritis can cause you not to function properly when taking care of your daily activities of living. Disfiguring may occur from joint damage.

There is no said cure for rheumatoid arthritis. Our goal in treating rheumatoid arthritis is to reduce the amount of inflammation you are suffering from to stop the progression of joint damage. I would like to discuss what is available today regarding medication to help the arthritic rheumatoid patient.

Nonsteroidal anti-inflammatory drugs reduce inflammation and relieve pain. There are versions over the counter like I mentioned before like Motrin and Aleve and stronger prescription versions like Celebrex, and Naprosyn. When these NSAIDs are repeatedly used the side effect profile becomes more prominent. Side effects include ringing of your ears, gastric ulcers, heart problems, stomach bleeding, and liver and kidney damage. If these medications are consumed with alcohol or taken with corticosteroids the risk of intestinal bleeding is greater.

Another alternative commonly used by your doctor is corticosteroid medication like prednisone and methylprednisolone (Medrol) which reduce inflammation and pain. In my clinical experience steroids make you feel better right away but when used for many years, they may become less effective and cause side effects. Side effects include thinning of the bones, easy bruising, weight gain, a round face and diabetes. Your doctor should gradually taper off the medication when he prescribes it over time.

If your rheumatoid arthritis is in it's early stages and your doctor wants to prevent further joint and tissue damage then he may prescribe Disease-Modifying Antirheumatic Drugs also known as DMARDs. You may need to take these drugs for months before you notice any benefit. The names of these medications are called Plaquenil, Gold Compounds, Ridaura, Sulfasalazine, Minocycline and Methotrexate.

When your arthritis is out of control and you need to tame your immune system there are drugs you can take called immunosuppressants. Some commonly used are leflunomide (Arava), azathioprine (Imuran), cyclosporine (Neoral), and cyclophosphamide (Cytoxan). These types of medications can contribute to serious infections in the body.

Other drugs are available today to treat rheumatoid arthritis. These drugs are called TNF-alpha inhibitors. These medications act like anti-inflammatory medicine that help reduce pain, morning stiffness and tender joints. Although they may take up to three weeks to take affect they may stop the progression of disease. These medications are often taken with Methotrexate. TNF inhibitors are Enbrel, Remicade, and Humira. Be aware that the side effect profile may be higher. Side effects include local irritation at the injection site, worsening of conjestive heart failure, blood disorders, increase potential for infection, lymphoma, demyelinating disease. If you ever have sign of any infection your doctor should never use these drugs!

For the patient who suffers from rheumatoid arthritis that is not helped thus far another class of medication exists which is called interleukin-1 receptor antagonist otherwise known as IL-1Ra. The name of this medication is called Anakinra or Kineret. You self administer this drug under the skin daily. These drugs are often given with Methotrexate also. The side effects of these drugs include irritation at the injection site, an increase in upper respiratory infections, headaches and increase in infections.

Newer treatments exists today with very good results. These include medications which inactivate your T cells in your immune system. These drugs reduce the inflammation and joint damage caused by rheumatoid arthritis. This treatment is usually reserved for patients who are not helped by TNF-alpha inhibitors. The name of this drug is called Orencia and is given monthly through a vein in your arm. Again side effects include headache, nausea, and pneumonia.

Now available to patients is the new drug called Rituxan which works by reducing the B cells in your body. B cell production is significant in the role of inflammation. This drug is usually given with Methotrexate. This drug is given in your vein also. Side effects include fever, chills and nausea. Rituxan has been associated and now linked to fatal brain infections.

Different surgical procedures have been performed to help the severe rheumatoid arthritic patients. Total joint replacement has been used with prosthesis, tendon repair has been done, and removing the lining of the joint has given relief to certain patients.

Understanding your type of rheumatoid arthritis and it's severity is the key factor. Using a combination of healthy diet, assistive devices, exercise program, medications available and knowing your limits all help in treating rheumatoid arthritis.

CHAPTER 4

GOUT

This type of arthritis is characterized by a sudden attack of pain which accompanies redness and tenderness of the joint being affected. When this happens you can be having an acute attack of gouty arthritis. Men are more likely to get gout attack than women. After menopause women can get gout more frequently.

The symptoms of gout usually affect the large joint of your big toe but can occur in your knees, hands, wrists, feet and ankles. Typically the pain can last for five to ten days and then completely resolves. In the meantime the joint that is affected can become red, hot and swollen.

Gout is known to occur when in your blood you develop high levels of uric acid which come from foods high in purines. These foods are organ meats, anchovies, hering, asparagus and mushrooms. Urate crystals then form when your body breaks down these excess purines. Normally, uric acid dissolves in your blood and passes through your kidneys into your urine. But sometimes your body either produces too much uric acid or your kidneys excrete too little uric acid. When this happens, uric acid can build up, forming sharp, needle-like urate crystals in a joint or surrounding tissue that cause pain, inflammation and swelling.

We now know that certain risk factor are present that increase the uric acid level in your body. Excessive alcohol use, usually more than two drinks a day increase your risk. There are certain types of medical conditions which when present increase your risk for gout. These conditions are high blood pressure or hypertension, diabetes, high levels of fat in your blood and arteriosclerosis which is narrowing of your arteries. In addition certain types of medication can cause and increase risk like the use of thiazide diuretics and low dose aspirin. Anti-rejection drugs used in organ transplants can cause a high uric acid in the blood. If your family has a history of gout then your risk increases.

When you go visit your doctor he may want to order some tests to confirm the diagnosis. A blood test to measure the amount of uric acid is important. Your doctor may want to exam the fluid taken from the joint to exam it for uratc crystals. These test can confirm the diagnosis. When a patient suffers from repeated attacks of gout then the deposit which form under the skin can cause nodules called tophi. During an attack the tophi can become painful to touch. If repeated attacks occur then it should be suggested by your doctor that medication can reduce the complication of forming kidney stones.

Certain medications are used in treating gout. The nonsteriodal anti-inflammatory drugs can be used. Colchicine is great to treat gout but has side effects. Nausea, vomiting and diarrhea are common. Another drug commonly used is Prednisone or steroids. If taken orally it is effective and can be given into the joint. If you suffer from repeated painful attacks per year then there are medications which are available to help prevent the attacks from coming back. Allopurinol can limit the amount of uric acid made in the body. The side effects from this medication include rashes on the skin and low blood counts. Probenecid will help remove uric acid from your body. Side effects of this medication include stomach pain and skin rashes.

Diet is also a treatment for gout. Cut back on the amount of red meat and seafood you eat. Avoid alcoholic beverages. Eat low fat dairy products. You can also eat more complex carbohydrates like whole grain breads. By following these simple instructions you will reduce your risk of getting an attack and treat subsequent attacks effectively.

CHAPTER 5

PSEUDOGOUT

Pseudogout is a form of arthritis which is characterized by painful swelling in one or more joints. The joint more commonly affected is the knee. Pseudogout is similar to gout. Like gout, pseudogout causes sudden, severe pain in a joint. Crystals form in the joint lining. The name is called pseudogout because a different kind of crystal is formed in the joint.

Pseudogout most commonly affects your knees, but can affect your ankles, hands, wrists, elbows and shoulders. Symptoms that are common are swelling of the affected joint, warmth over the joint affected and severe joint pain.

The type of crystal identified in the lining of the joint is called calcium pyrophosphate. The crystals form in the cartilage in and around your joints. We do not know why it occurs. When deposits form from this disease it can also cause calcification of joint cartilage called chondrocalcinosis. It can also cause joint degeneration.

There are certain risk factor for the disease. Older adults are more prone to the disease. Having joint replacement surgery or trauma to your joint increases your risk of developing crystals. Families with genetic disorders like Familial Chondrocalcinosis develop pseudogout. Excess iron can be stored in your organs and tissues around your joints called hemochromatosis. These patients also have pseudogout development.

If you present to your doctor with these symptoms your doctor may have to draw blood. Because gout and pseudogout can present with similar symptoms analyzing the joint fluid can help the doctor make the proper diagnosis. He then will look under a microscope to see the calcium crystals and confirm the diagnosis is pseudogout. He may want to take

X-rays. By doing this he can see the joint cartilage will be calcified.

Complications from pseudogout include joint damage, bone cysts, bone spurs and cartilage loss. When treating a patient with pseudogout you want to treat the pain and inflammation. Nonsteroidal drugs like Motrin, and prescription Indocin will reduce the amount of inflammation. Another choice includes Colchicine. Often in my practice I would give an injection of corticosteroids after aspirating the joint. Like all treatments one must discuss the alternative treatments in conjunction with therapy offered to give the patient proper relief.

CHAPTER 6

PSORIATIC ARTHRITIS

People who develop psoriasis of the skin are more likely to get psoriatic arthritis of the joints. You may develop joint stiffness and swelling. Any part of your body can be affected. There is currently no cure for psoriatic arthritis.

Often skin and joint problems appear and disappear at the same time. Both of these diseases could be chronic. The symptoms that appear are swollen joints that are tender to touch associated with various degrees of pain. There are five types of psoriatic arthritis that you may experience.

Asymmetric psoriatic arthritis is the mildest form which usually affects one side of your body or different joints on each side. Fewer than five joints are involved. If the tendons cause your fingers and toes to become swollen and tender then your fingers and toes resemble a sausage shape. The medical term for this is called dactylitis. If the psoriasis is severe then you usually present with arthritis on one side. Usually five or more joints are affected on the same side of your body. This condition affects more women than men. Another type of psoriatic arthritis that affects mostly men is called distal interphalangeal joint involvement. This condition is named for the joints it affects. Joints like the finger, toes and nails could be affected. The nail itself shows signs of thickening and pitting. When we refer to the spine we called it spondylitis. Areas most affected are your lower back, neck and sacroiliac joints. As this disease progresses movement becomes more restricted and painful. The last most disabling form of the disease is called Psoriatic Mutilans. In this condition you get a painful and disabling form of the disease. As time progresses with the disease the small bones in the hands become destroyed.

When we discuss causes we now know that psoriasis is a skin condition with a rapid buildup of rough, dry, dead skin that form into thick scales. The arthritic component causes pain and stiffness in our joints. Both of these conditions are autoimmune causes. This means that your body begins to attack healthy tissue and cells. When this inflammation takes place it causes inflammation in the joints that cause an overproduction of skin cells to be produced. Many people with psoriatic arthritis have a relative with the disease and researchers have found certain genetic markers appear to be associated with psoriatic arthritis. Another cause for psoriatic arthritis is due to physical trauma or something in the environment. This may be related to getting a previous bacterial or viral infection. In people who develop psoriatic arthritis a substance called tumor necrosis factor causes inflammation in rheumatoid arthritis. People with psoriatic arthritis have high levels of tumor necrosis factor in both their joints and skin.

Having psoriatic arthritis can be painful and debilitating, and can damage a joint. Psoriatic arthritis can cause painful fingers and toes. Often when this happens it is hard to fit shoes properly so you may need to see a podiatrist for special shoes. Associated with psoriatic arthritis is enthesopathy which causes pain at the point where the ligaments and tendons attach to bones. There is an increase in the amount of cases of Achilles Tendonitis and in Plantar Faciitis and inflammation to the bottom of your foot. Neck and back pain also can happen. Due to psoriatic arthritis a condition called Spondylitis can occur. This condition causes inflammation of the joints between the vertebrae of your spine and the joints between your spine and pelvis.

When you have the possibility of having psoriatic arthritis test help make the diagnosis. X-rays help see the changes in the joints that occur in psoriatic arthritis. Examining the synovial fluid will help rule in or out the diagnosis. Doing a blood test called the sedimentation rate will tell if your body is inflamed.

No treatment exist for psoriatic arthritis so we try to control the amount of inflammation you have and by doing this you will feel better and ultimately you will have less pain and joint destruction. Drugs such as aspirin and ibuprofen may help control pain, swelling and morning stiffness. Also nonsteriodal drugs will help. Corticosteroid oral medication or injections may help control the inflammation. Using disease –modifying drugs like Asulfidine and Methorexate have not only stopped the inflammation but has shown to stop the destruction of the joints.

Another treatment to stop your immune system from harming itself in this disease is the medications called immunosuppressant drugs. Using these drugs have shown to stop your immune system from attacking healthy tissue with people suffering from psoriatic arthritis. Immunosuppressant drugs include Imuran , Arava and Neoral. Because these are reserved for the more severe cases the side effect potential is greater. These drugs suppress the immune system and can cause anemia, and increased risk for infection. Liver and kidney damage has also been reported. That is why it is essential to have your doctor take routine blood test to monitor these values.

If your doctor feels that your psoriatic arthritis is very severe there is a new treatment called tumor necrosis factor-alpha inhibitors. When given these medications protein will be blocked that cause inflammation. Drugs in this category are named Enbrel, Humira, and Remicade. Keep in mind that this treatment is administered intravenously and is costly. Check with your insurance company about coverage before starting it.

Surgery too is an alternative if the joints are disfiguring and restrict mobility. New alternative medication will be discussed later on in this book.

CHAPTER 7

LUPUS

Another type of arthritis that is an inflammatory type that attacks your immune system is called lupus. Lupus is considered a systemic disease which means that it can affect many different body systems, including your joints, skin, kidneys, blood cells and your heart and lungs. Women are now affected more than men. Years ago the outcome for lupus was not good but today we have made many advances which make the treatment and understanding of lupus a treatable disease.

Lupus patients present differently. Signs and symptoms may come suddenly or develop slowly. In my practice I would usually see patients when they were "flaring up" or get worsening signs and symptoms. There are many different

kinds of signs and symptoms which people present with. Fatigue, fever, weight loss or gain, lesions of the skin which get worse with sun exposure, joint pain, stiffness and swelling are common. A butterfly rash which we call malar rash can appear on your cheeks and nose. Mouth sores, hair loss, shortness of breath may appear. Your fingers and toes can turn blue when exposed to cold or during stressful periods. Chest pain and dry eyes and easy bruising can be present. Anxiety, depression and memory loss occurs frequently.

Although we do not know what actually causes lupus we know it is an immune disease which turns against our healthy tissue in our body. When the inflammation happens damage occurs to different parts of our body including the joints, skin, kidneys, heart, lungs, and blood vessels and brain. People who develop lupus may have an inherited gene. Lupus is said to be triggered by different kinds of medication and viruses.

There are four known types of lupus. Each has their own prognosis and treatment. The first type known is systemic lupus erythematosus which can affect any part of your body. The typical body systems often affected are the skin, joints, lungs, kidney, and blood. This is the most common type of lupus. Discoid lupus erythematosus affects the skin and is also called cutaneous lupus. People present with a rash on the face, neck or scalp. Drug-induced lupus erythematosus occurs from certain prescription drugs. Neonatal lupus is the fourth and most rare. This affects newborn babies. Mothers often pass certain antibodies to their blood. A newborn may have a rash within weeks of being born.

You may increase your risk for lupus if you are a female and if your age is between 15 and 30 years old. Lupus is more common in blacks and in Asians. Sunlight may trigger an internal response in people. Certain prescription drugs can potentially trigger lupus. The medications which now have proven to trigger lupus include the antipsychotic drug chlorpromazine, high blood pressure medication, and procainamide. It should be said that it may take several months for these drugs to cause lupus. It is also known that patients who have been infected with the common virus Epstein-Barr are more prone to develop lupus. New data suggest that certain chemical exposure to silica and mercury make patients more likely to develop lupus.

It is difficult even today to diagnose lupus. The American College of Rheumatology has developed eleven criteria that lupus patients have. If you have four of these criteria then you will be diagnosed with lupus. The eleven criteria are as follows: a rash on the face called a malar rash, a scaly rash called a discoid rash which has raised scaly patches, a sun exposed rash, mouth sores, joint pain or swelling in two or more joints, kidney disease, seizures, low blood counts, or low platelet counts, a positive anti-nuclear antibody tests, or a positive double-stranded anti-DNA test.

When lupus is finally diagnosed it is important for your doctor to make sure that complications do not occur. For example if the kidneys become damaged they will not function and cause death. If the nervous system is affected a patient may experience, headaches, dizziness, memory problems, behavior changes and even seizures. When the lungs become inflamed pleurisy can develop which will give you pain when taking a deep breath. If the heart becomes inflamed the muscle will be affected called myocarditis. Arteries can become inflamed called arteritis. New studies reveal a correlation between lung cancer and non-Hodgkin's lymphoma. Avascular necrosis is another complication when blood supply to the bone diminishes. Finally the risk of pregnancy complications are higher. Lupus increases the risk of high blood pressure and preterm birth.

In treating lupus we want to see the signs and symptoms. When your signs and symptoms are mild to moderate we start treatment with the nonsteroidal anti-infammatory drugs. Drugs like Naprosyn are used. Antimalarial drugs are used like Plaquenil may prevent flares of the disease. Be aware of the side effects of Plaquenil like vision problems and muscle weakness. Using corticosteroids have also helped the inflammation in lupus. If lupus presents with more aggressive symptoms a higher dose of steroids may be given. Always have your doctor remind you of the side effect profile of corticosteroids which is infection, mood swings, high blood pressure and osteoporosis. Drugs that suppress the immune system may help. These medications include Cytoxan and Imuran. Combinations of the drugs have also been used and may be successful.

CHAPTER 8

SCLERODERMA

A progressive disease which involves hardening of the connective tissues of the body and skin tightening is called scleroderma. There are two main types known today. Localized scleroderma involves the skin only. Systemic scleroderma can involve the heart, lungs, kidneys, and digestive tract. Scleroderma is considered a rare disease which can affect approximately 250 people per million. Scleroderma has been prevalent in families with known scleroderma.

There are common symptoms to both types of disease. A patient may present with raynaud's phenomenon. This is a condition where small blood vessels constrict in the hands and feet causing numbness and color changes of the toes and fingers. Patients often have gastroesophageal reflux which can damage the section of the esophagus nearest the stomach. You may notice a tightening of the skin around the mouth, face and fingers.

In localized scleroderma you will find oval shaped thickened patches of skin called morphea. In children mostly you can get linear scleroderma which features bands of hardened skin in the legs and arms. If you are diagnosed with systemic scleroderma then not only is your skin involved but your blood vessels and internal organs can be affected.

It is known today that scleroderma results from an overproduction of collagen in the body tissues. This is the substance that holds your skin and connective tissues together. The immune system is also affected and the body produces inflammation.

Race and sex play a role with scleroderma. The Native Americans in Oklahoma are at twenty times the risk for developing scleroderma. In addition we now know that systemic scleroderma is more common in African Americans. Women are four times more likely to get scleroderma than men. New research has discovered that silica dust, solvents like paint thinners, and chemotherapy agents can cause scleroderma.

When a physician sees these changes it is harder to treat these patients and the more aggressive he has to treat the patient. Complications can be a severe form of Raynaud's disease. Because of the restricted blood flow to the fingertips damage to the tissue occurs causing ulcers in the flesh. In some cases gangrene and amputation can result from the damaged tissue. In the lung when scar tissue results you lose the capacity to expand the lungs properly which results in pulmonary fibrosis. Also when the pulmonary arteries become restricted from fibrosis you may get pulmonary hypertension. If the kidney become affected you will see elevated protein in the urine which results in hypertension and kidney failure. When the heart itself is affected scarring occurs which can cause arrthymias (abnormal heart beats) and fluid to build up in the lungs called conjestive heart failure. Also if the lining surrounding the heart becomes inflamed this is called pericarditis. Dental complications occur because the mouth becomes smaller and narrower. People with scleroderma do not produce normal amounts of saliva. Because of this their risk of decay is greater. As an end result teeth may become loose and fall out. Men who develop scleroderma experience erectile dysfunction. Scleroderma can also affect women by decreasing sexual lubrication and constricting the vaginal opening.

When a doctor evaluates you for scleroderma he will obtain certain blood tests to evaluate the immune system. Certain antibodies are usually elevated. A doctor will also in certain cases do a biopsy of the affected skin to see abnormalities in the skin.

There is no cure for the overproduction of collagen. The goal in treatment is to stop the symptoms and prevent complications. Medications that dilate blood vessels will help the lung and kidneys and help Raynaud's disease. Taking drugs to suppress the immune system will help the overall symptoms.

In treating the scleroderma patient, physical therapy will help strength and mobility and improve pain to maintain your daily activities of living. Treating skin lesions with exposure to ultraviolet light may be beneficial. Laser surgery may help the skin lesions.

An end result from scleroderma of the fingertips is gangrene. If this is present then amputation may be necessary. Lung transplants have been done if the lung arteries develop hypertension. Other measures like protecting yourself from the cold would also be recommended.

CHAPTER 9

LYME DISEASE

Lyme disease is transmitted by a tick that causes signs and symptoms from rash, fever, chills and body aches to joint swelling. It has been known to cause weakness and temporary paralysis. The disease is caused by bacteria Borrelia Burgdorferi. The deer tick can feed on humans or animals. Lyme disease can affect any part of your body.

The tick bite starts out with redness and expands. It can be as small as a penny or as large as a dollar bill. It often looks like a target with a central clearing. The name of the rash is Erythema Migrans. But not everyone gets the rash. It affects about 80% of the people. A patient may develop flu like symptoms and give the patient fever, fatigue, body aches, and headache. You may develop severe joint pain and swelling several months after the infection takes place. One of the most common joints affected is the knee. Neurological symptoms may occur too. The meningis (the membranes surrounding your brain) may be affected, and you may develop Bell's Palsy, which is a numbness on one side of your face. A patient may experience weakness of your limbs and memory loss. A late finding is heart problems. An irregular heart beat, eye inflammation and hepatitis are reported too.

Lyme disease is caused by the bacteria Borrelia Burgdorferi carried by the deer tick. When the deer tick feeds off the blood of it's host it engorges it's size. At the time the tick feeds off the blood of it's hosts the bacteria is transferred to the hosts which starts the infection process. Deer ticks are most active in the summer. Removing a tick as soon as it is attached to your skin may prevent the disease or infection.

There are certain risks in getting Lyme disease. Avoid spending time in wooded or grassy areas. In the United States the most prevalent place to find deer tick is in the Northeast and Midwest regions. If you are in areas which have known ticks wear long sleeve clothing.

If you see your doctor with these familiar symptoms your doctor will order some blood tests to confirm the diagnosis. The test which often detects Lyme disease is called the Elisa test which stands for Enzyme-linked immunosorbent assay test. This test detects antibodies to the bacteria. When this test is positive the Western blot test confirms the diagnosis. If you wanted to diagnose Lyme disease in an infected joint you would order the Polymerase Chain Reaction Test which detects the bacterial DNA in the infected fluid.

Sometimes it is difficult to detect that a patient has lyme disease because of all the different symptoms and complications a patient can present with. The complications of untreated lyme disease can be chronic joint inflammation, neurological symptoms like neuropathy, impaired memory, heart rhythm irregularities, and changes in sleep habits.

The treatment for early-stage lyme disease is oral antibiotics. The regime is doxycycline for adults and children older than 8, or amoxicillin for adults, or pregnant women. Usually the treatment is for 14-21 day course. In my practice we have also seen patients presenting with advanced symptoms and complications. These patients received intravenous antibiotics for 14 to 28 days. But the way to treat the disease is to avoid it. Use a repellent with 10 to 30 percent DEET concentration. The amount of DEET used is determined by the length of time spent exposed. One of the biggest misconceptions is once you have had lyme disease you cannot get it again is not true. You can be re-infected again!

CHAPTER 10

FIBROMYALGIA

Often for the doctor and patient I have found fibromyalgia one of the most frustrating conditions to treat. Fibromyalgia occurs in just 2% of the population in the United States. Women develop the disorder more than men and as you get older the risk for the disease gets higher.

Fibromyalgia is a condition with widespread pain in your ligament, tendons, and muscles which give you multiple areas of tender points on your body. You also become very fatigued. What is interesting is that your doctor will give you tests to determine what is the problem and all of the testing will be negative. So the diagnosis ends up being one of exclusion. Patients have described the pain as a constant dull ache of the muscles. But the pain must occur on both sides of your body which give you tender points to touch. The most common points are the back of the head, between the shoulder blades, top of the shoulders, outer elbows, sides of the hips, inner part of the knees, and the upper chest. The patients have sleep disturbances and sleep apnea.

Conditions associated with fibromyalia include depression, chronic fatigue syndrome, endometriosis, headaches, irritable bowl syndrome, rheumatoid arthritis, post-traumatic stress disorder, lupus, osteoarthritis, and restless leg syndrome.

We do not know for sure what causes fibromyalgia but there are a variety of factors which contribute to the condition. Infections may aggravate or trigger fibromyalgia. Having a family member may make you more susceptible to get the condition. Any sort of trauma or stress related disorder has been linked to fibromyalgia.

It is now known that people with fibromalgia have a lower threshold for pain because there is increased sensitivity in the brain to pain signals. The brain's receptors seem to develop memory of the pain and become sensitive and overreact to pain signals.

Because of the difficulty establishing and making a diagnosis of fibromyalgia The American College of Rheumatology has established two criteria for the diagnosis of fibromyalgia. One is at least 11 positive tender points out of a total of 18 and widespread pain which lasts at least 3 months.

In testing for the condition your doctor will order a ESR test, thyroid function tests and complete blood count to rule out other common conditions. When treating this condition after it has been established medications can help reduce the amount of pain and also improve sleep. Medications like analgesics, Tylenol, nonsteroidal anti-inflammatory medications, antidepressants, and anti-seizure medication can be useful. In addition physical therapy can restore muscle balance and reduce pain. Counseling with behavioral therapy can help you deal with stressful situations. Try to get enough sleep, and maintain a healthy lifestyle will help the overall condition.

CHAPTER 11

CARPAL TUNNEL SYNDROME

I have included a chapter on carpal tunnel syndrome because of how common the condition is and because of the many common causes that have now known to cause it. The carpal tunnel located at the wrist is a narrow passageway which is located specifically on the palm side of your wrist. The tunnel protects a main nerve to your hand and nine tendons that make your fingers bend. When any pressure is placed on the nerve your get numbness, pain, and weakness which is known as carpal tunnel syndrome.

When the symptom first starts it will cause a gradual aching in your wrist and forearm. You may experience a tingling or numbness of your thumb and index finger, middle or ring finger but not your little finger. These symptoms occur when you wake up from sleep or can occur while holding an object, steering wheel, or phone.

The causes of carpal tunnel syndrome is due to a pressure on the median nerve. The median nerve provides sensation to the fingers and muscle motor function. So when the nerve is affected you lose sensation and motor function. There are reasons as to why you develop median nerve pressure resulting in carpal tunnel syndrome. Rheumatoid arthritis, and diabetes, thyroid disorders and menopause can cause carpal tunnel syndrome. Pregnancy and amyloidosis can cause carpal tunnel syndrome. Repetitive flexing and extending of the tendons in the hands and wrists can increase pressure within the carpal tunnel.

One risk factor to develop carpal tunnel syndrome is your sex. Women are three times likely as men to develop carpal tunnel syndrome. Hereditary factors like the shape of your wrist, or close relatives who have the problem are more likely to develop carpal tunnel syndrome. People with end stage kidney disease can develop it.

When I suspected a patient of having carpal tunnel syndrome there are two common test ordered to confirm the diagnosis. One test is called the electromyogram test. This test measures the electrical charges produced by muscles. This test accesses for muscle damage. Another test is the nerve conduction test. A small shock is passed through the median nerve to see if electrical impulses are slowed in the carpal tunnel.

The treatment of carpal syndrome with mild symptoms would be to take more frequent breaks from doing the repetitive motion. You can apply cold compress to the swelling area. A wrist splint will stop the wrist from movement which may be aggravating the wrist. Nonsteroidal anti-inflammatory drugs may help relieve pain form carpal tunnel syndrome. If the symptoms persist then corticosteroids may be injected to reduce the inflammation.

A consensus among doctors if all else fails and you have continued symptoms for more than six months then surgery can be performed releasing the affected nerve.

CHAPTER 12

PLANTAR FASCIITIS

Plantar fasciitis is a very common cause of heel pain. The plantar fascia connects your heel bone to your toes. It is a thick band of tissue. When you have plantar fasciitis you may get a pain when you get up in the morning which is described as knifelike. People who run commonly develop plantar fasciitis. People who are overweight, pregnant patients, and patients who have inadequate shoes usually develop plantar fasciitis.

Common symptoms are pain under the foot. The pain is usually of one foot but can develop to both feet. The pain has been described as heel pain. Risk factors for plantar fasciitis include age. Plantar fasciitis most commonly occurs between the ages of 40 to 60. Women are more likely than men to develop plantar fasciitis. Ballet dancers, or any type of exercise which puts an extra strain on your joints. Being flat footed or having a high arch can predispose plantar fasciitis. Obesity is a risk factor.

When a doctor today suspects plantar fasciitis your doctor will order an MRI to make sure that you do not have another problem like a stress fracture of the foot which presents clinically the same way. Medications like non-steroidal anti-infammatory drugs help the symptoms. Corticosteroids can be used also. Physical therapy can give you stretching exercises which should help you in the morning. Other treatments include a splint fitted to your calf and foot while you sleep. This holds the plantar fascia and Achilles tendon in a lengthened position overnight so that they can be stretched effectively. Doctors will often prescribe orthotics to distribute the pressure of the arch more evenly. New in treatment is extracorporeal shock wave therapy. This involves sound waves directed at the area of the heel to stimulate healing. Lastly surgery has been used to detach from the heel bone the plantar fascia. One can also try to do more low impact exercises and maintain a healthy weight.

CHAPTER 13

ALTERNATIVE MEDICATION TREATMENTS

In this chapter I will discuss alternative treatments and medication to treating your arthritic pain and inflammation. Today doctors who have treated his or her patient have looked into treating their patients with alternative supplements and procedures. I would highly recommend that before treating yourself with these methods or supplements discuss with your treating doctor before starting as you do not want to interfere with your current medications or treatment.

Acupuncture done by a reputable practitioner has given the patient more short term relief from pain than long term.

The studies show that the needles that are inserted redirect your body's energy in order to relieve pain.

Ginger extract now has shown to reduce pain in osteoarthritis. It should be noted that ginger should not be taken with coumadin a blood thinner. Ginger has also been reported to cause heartburn and diarrhea.

Glucosamine and chondroitin have been beneficial with people with osteoarthritis. Note that glucosamine should not be taken if you are allergic to shellfish. Chondroitin Sulfate may also affect the dosage of coumadin. Magnets a safe treatment is worn near the painful joint. Patients of mine have had significant relief from magnet therapy.

There are alternative treatments for rheumatoid arthritis too. New studies released confirm that plant oils that contain gamma-linolenic acid or GLA can help with pain and morning stiffness. GLA is a type of omega- 6 fatty acid that comes from plant oils, such as primrose, borage and black currant. Side effects include nausea, diarrhea and gas.

Fish oil that contains eicosapentaenoic acid (EPA) or

docosahexaenoic acid (DHA) are omega-3 fatty acids found in fish oil. These supplements have been found to reduce the amount of inflammation in patients with rheumatoid arthritis. Side effects include belching, and nausea.

Gout too has had alternative treatments. There has now been a clear association with people who drink coffee and gout attacks. Researchers have found that coffee drinkers whether caffeinated or non-caffeinated drinkers have had a higher incidence in the severity of gout attacks.

Supplements containing vitamin C may reduce the levels of uric acid in your blood. Increase your intake of vitamin C by eating fruits and vegetables, especially oranges. Cherries, blackberries, blueberries, purple grapes, and raspberries have been shown to lower the levels of uric acid.

Alternative medication has been used to treat psoriatic arthritis. Long term studies have shown that a carotenoid called beta-cryptoxanthin and the mineral zinc may help prevent some forms of arthritis. Beta-cryptoxanthin is a substance found in fruits and vegetables and is converted in your body into retinol which is an active form of vitamin A. You can get this supplement from papaya, red bell peppers, oranges, corn and watermelon. Foods that are rich in zinc include liver, sesame and pumpkin seeds, yogurt and shrimp.

Today we now know that a diet which contains cruciferous vegetables like broccoli, cauliflower, brussel sprouts is associated with a reduced risk of arthritis. It is also thought that glucosamine and chondroitin supplements help the body repair cartilage damaged by arthritis and may relieve pain and treat psoriasis. Fish oil supplements reduce arthritic pain, swelling and stiffness as they are known to enhance the effectiveness of anti-inflammatory medication.

In treating lupus with new alternative medication you want to try to build the immune system so you can prevent lupus from getting worse. One procedure that is now being introduced is stem cell transplant. This uses your own stem cells to rebuild your immune system. This is now being used for life- threatening cases of lupus. The hormone dehyhdroepiandrosterone or DHEA has been shown in clinical trials to improve the quality of life in people with lupus. Rituximab has been used to decrease B cells in your body to help them fight off lupus. Note that this drug has caused fatal infections. For lupus patients fish oil has shown some promise with lupus patients and taking flaxseed which contains a fatty acid called alpha-linolenic acid which can decrease the bodies inflammation.

Success has been given to patients who have had been given Vitamin B6. Relief has been shown in clinical trials. Ultrasound treatments may also be used and has shown to help patients.

Bromelain (from pineapple) is an enzyme that helps heal tissue and speed up the removal of inflammatory waste products from the joint.

Papain from Papaya can also be helpful. Tumeric of curcumin, which is known as a spice is a powerful anti-inflammatory that works as well as cortisone for some people.

As you can see there is a lot of research that is currently going on now to improve these diseases. Used whenever feasible with other treatments has been shown to be successful overall when treating different kinds of arthritis.

CHAPTER 14

AVOID FOODS THAT TRIGGER ARTHRITIS

If you are one of the millions of people who suffer from arthritis this chapter may be one of the most important chapters you will read. I have used over 25 years of hearing patients why they have "flare-ups" and what they have been eating prior to their "flare-up" and there have been remarkable consistencies in patients stories and histories.

We know today that allergies can be triggered from various foods and the latest new data and research have proven that arthritis inflammation can also be triggered from certain foods. As a practicing physician I have repeatedly confirmed this data. In certain cases there are foods which will trigger an acute flare up or exacerbate one's symptoms.

Any food which is believed to promote inflammation or increase pain is considered a food or food group to avoid. Salt will trigger any type of inflammation to the affected joint and will make the process of healing delayed due to the retention of unwanted fluid exacerbated by salt in the joint. Dairy products have been proven to trigger arthritis inflammation. The heavier the cream the worse the symptoms. Red meat has been shown to increase the inflammatory process. Today we now know that there are four leading vegetables which can trigger the inflammatory process which result in pain. These vegetables are eggplant, bell peppers, tomatoes, and potatoes. Excess sugar and sour fruits should be eliminated. In addition wine and cheese could exacerbate arthritis. It is believed that the more you eat in quantity has a direct correlation with your exacerbation and duration of the flare up. Some patients have seen an immediate improvement in their symptoms once these foods are eliminated. You can try this yourself by strictly eliminating them from your diet for a two to three week period and then see how you feel. It is important to state that you should not eliminate an entire food group without consulting with your physician as this could have serious consequences with your entire health.

If diagnosed with gout, foods that have purines should be avoided. Foods that should be avoided are hot dogs, bacon, game foods, chicken and turkey. Shellfish, shrimp, salmon have been shown to trigger an acute gout attack. Alcohol when ingested in excessive amounts can trigger an attack. Beer has been noted to have more purines than alcohol. Legumes can cause a problem for the gout patient.

Your body metabolizes purines into uric acid. When this acid gets out of control it settles in your joints and causes painful gout. It should also be noted that a diet high in sodium content can cause dehydration which can trigger an attack too.

So as you can see there are many foods that you should try to avoid or at least eat in moderation to see if this could improve your outcome of alleviating pain and inflammation.